EMANUELE M. BARBONI DALLA COSTA

Answers on Love, Relationships and Emotional Communication

Contents

Introduction   vi

 1 GENERATE ATTRACTION   1

 2 How do you overcome shyness with girls?   2

 3 What's the first thing women look at in a man?   6

 4 What makes a person interesting and attractive?   9

 5 What's your favorite way to show some-
     one you care?   12

 6 Can you recommend daily exercises I can
     do to improve my...   13

 7 Why do people talk even when they don't
     know the topic being...   17

 8 LOVE AND RELATIONSHIPS   19

 9 What can we do to limit misunderstand-
     ings in relationships?   20

10 How to get over unrequited love?   22

11 If a girl writes to a guy all day, does that
     mean she's in...   25

12 The girl I have a crush on says she likes
     me but won't...   27

13 How can I "destroy" an idealized love?   30

14 How to manage a relationship with a colleague? 32

15 What to do if you are in love with a girl,
     but haven't...   34

16 What does it mean if someone who loves
    you ignores you and...   36
17 What's one "man problem" that women
    wouldn't understand?   39
18 FIRST DATE   42
19 What do you think would be the ideal
    place for a first date?   43
20 How not to look "desperate" on a first date   46
21 How to impress a girl on a first date?   48
22 What not to do on a first date?   50
23 What to say to a girl after a first date?   52
24 What should you know before you kiss someone?   54
25 Does there have to be physical contact
    on the first date?   56
26 BETTER CONVERSATIONS   59
27 What does a good conversation consist of?   60
28 What is the best way to start an online conversation?   63
29 How do you start a conversation?   66
30 How can you keep the level of conversa-
    tion up?   68
31 What's the best way to get out of a con-
    versation where...   71
32 How can I improve my public speaking skills?   74
33 BREAKING UP AND TAKING BACK   75
34 I want to break up with my girlfriend.
    What are the best...   76
35 My boyfriend and I have picked up and
    broken up several...   78
36 What does it mean if she likes me a lot
    but wants to be...   79
37 Is love there when you miss your partner?   81

38 Can true love be at first sight?   84
39 Why do some people when they break
    up immediately look for...   86
40 OVERCOMING THE FEAR OF TALK-
    ING TO PEOPLE   90
41 I'm a boring person, how can I change?   91
42 How to deal with people who only talk
    about themselves?   93
43 Why is it that when you try to speak or
    enter a...   97
44 What to do when you have difficulty
    talking to people?   100
The Author   103
Resources   105

Introduction

During my coaching sessions I was often faced with recurring questions. Many, many learners showed that they had the same criticality, the same doubt, the same uncertainty.

Thus the idea for this book was born: a collection of my students' "frequently asked questions" (and their answers).

Thus was born this book, in its version 1.0, with the intention of being useful to many of you and with the hope of clarifying many points in relation to the relationship you have with yourself and with others.

1

GENERATE ATTRACTION

2

How do you overcome shyness with girls?

There is a method to **overcoming shyness with girls**, and you won't find it in any seduction manual or online tutorial.

I'll reveal this in a moment, but it's necessary to back up a little first.

Underlying the emotion of shyness reside two **enormous fears**: that of **judgment** and that of **rejection**.

These are *"primordial"* fears, common to all human beings and capable of governing enormous social nuclei. I speak of social nuclei because we cannot avoid thinking about the social context when we talk about shyness.

That's right: shyness is generated by society.

Imagine waking up, with no memory, on a desert island (a beautiful island, full of beautiful girls, also with no

memory or "social" reminiscence). Virgin minds, like Adam and Eve in the Garden of Eden.

When you first meet one of them, how would you act?

Would you be shy?

Of course not!

Your behavior would be **similar to that of an animal**, somewhere between curious and afraid.

But there wouldn't be any **shyness**, would there?

Since social rules (rightly) rule the world, **it's completely natural to feel these kinds of emotions** when we have to interact with someone else. So don't make a big deal out of it, take it easy because you're not alone!

But let's get to the heart of the matter: **you are not shy, you are "simply" afraid of being judged or rejected.**

Shyness, as I often tell my students during my professional coaching sessions on improving interpersonal communication, is almost always an **excuse for not taking action**.

So let's start with this assumption: **you're not shy**, you're afraid of the **consequences** an approach might have.

The good news is that my experience has led me to firmly maintain that **the "catastrophic" vision that is generated**

in your mind when you think about approaching someone is simply **HILARIOUS**.

Here's the thing: **what, on balance, can REALLY justify this fear of yours?**

- *Have you ever tried to approach a girl?*
- *What happened?*
- *Did he bite you?*
- *Did she turn into a giant seven-headed snake?*

I don't think so. Because shyness is based on assumptions, not hard facts (not always at least).

I know that what you imagine in your mind is catastrophic, but the only **valuable advice I want to give you today is this: be rational and evaluate in a concrete way the reaction the girls had** when you tried to approach them.

Don't exaggerate. Try to be objective.

We are social beings, we communicate to exist and here I want to give you **another tip, very important and really shocking** (if they had told me when I was young I would have taken many more opportunities):

When someone you just met rejects you, they are not judging you, they are judging the way you communicate.

That's right. He's not rejecting you but your way of communicating.

Every day I help my students to improve their interpersonal communication with my coaching programs and one of the first "walls" that I have to break through with them is precisely that of shyness.

The moment they realize

1. *the consequences of a "failed" approach are not as catastrophic as they thought and*
2. *that the rejection is not directed at them as individuals but at their communication*

they begin to understand that shyness can be defeated and real results can be achieved even if they are not experts.

You just need to be honest with yourself and in case get help from someone with experience!

3

What's the first thing women look at in a man?

The most unique ingredient that women notice in men is their **ability to converse and arouse emotions through the stories they tell about themselves.**

The field of communication is very broad and the question rather general, but I have not read in any answer that **refers to the ability of a man to entertain a woman verbally by telling her stories.**

To be more precise, I invite you to imagine a blind **date, a speed date for example, and take it as a specific case.**

In the first instance, a woman will observe the **physical** and **aesthetic appearance of** the man, trying to grasp also **olfactory and in general sensory elements** related to body language and para-verbal.

This is taught in any beginner's communication textbook, and has such a general foundation that it doesn't even come close to being a useful element.

This is an **initial screening of a purely aesthetic kind**. I'm not saying it doesn't count, on the contrary, but at this table where two strangers meet for the first time the situation still needs to "*warm up*".

Remember that the speed date only lasts ten minutes!

After the first **two minutes of** pleasantries and mutual observation (visual and sensory) we will begin to discuss, **introduce ourselves** and **tell something about ourselves**, right?

And this is where I think **the ability to tell your story can really make the difference** between a lucky *speed date* and a disastrous one.

The man can be as handsome as you like, but if as soon as he opens his mouth he is not able to involve or deal with topics of an insane banality, you can be sure that the female counterpart will run like hell.

Being able to tell **engaging stories, convey your values** through our phrases and **create emotional tension** are the elements I encourage you to focus on when dealing with a woman.

A woman also values a **man's listening skills** very highly, so learning how to properly handle **quality dialogue** is an absolutely necessary skill to break through.

Long story short: women look (like everyone else) at physical appearance, but they get involved for a man who can listen to them and move them.

4

What makes a person interesting and attractive?

In my experience what makes a person interesting is **their life story**.

That's right.

Everyone likes stories.

Because we're made of stories.

If you think about it, we are all protagonists of small and big daily adventures. We all have funny **anecdotes** to tell, **life stories** to share.

They can be nostalgic tales as well as funny, about challenge as well as growth.

Never underestimate the power of a story.

Our daily lives are a constant challenge, and we are all small but indomitable heroes.

An exam passed by the skin of your teeth, an addictive summer romance, a special moment of solitude, a moment of growth, a crazy night out with friends.

We all have small and big stories to tell.

Because everyone is **special**.

And our stories tell about who we are, the challenges we've faced, the projects we have in our drawer.

We all have that friend who when he talks about his life manages to charm the audience, right?

As you may have noticed, he never talks about great deeds, but about everyday matters. Rather mundane, really.

Yet we stand there, open-mouthed, waiting for the ending of this or that story.

That friend has a special gift: he **knows how to enhance his person through his stories.**

He manages to convey his values through the small and big challenges he has faced, and he manages to do so in an engaging way because he knows the art of storytelling and **manages to make even the story of the Wednesday bachelor-team match** with his colleagues an **engaging one.**

There, in my opinion without trying to be too clever or having to make up breathtaking stories **this is the characteristic that makes a person interesting**.

Don't just tell me you play *Magic*.

Tell me about how you started, why you started, what it felt like when you won your first game.

And make me excited.

Because you can be a person like any other but who can tell about himself, his world and his values with his little big stories.

5

What's your favorite way to show someone you care?

I have three favorite ways to show someone that I care about him or her.

1. **I listen to her with attention**. I show interest in her life, in her projects and I never fail to make my presence felt at important moments.
2. **I give them my time.** Time is the most precious resource we have and therefore it must be spared. If I care about a person you can tell immediately because I never fail to spend much of my precious time with them.
3. **I verbalize my feelings**. I tell him I care about her. Always, as soon as I get a chance. How many times have I missed the opportunity to say "I love you" because of insecurity or distraction. These small gestures may seem trivial but they make all the difference in so many people's lives.

6

Can you recommend daily exercises I can do to improve my charisma and be more confident?

Feeling "clumsy" is a fairly common criticism, but with a little practice your **communication** and **charisma** can **improve** in **no time**.

Here's my list of tips:

1. **Dress well**. You need to feel comfortable in the clothing you wear. Always try to have an eye for your style and make sure that it reflects your personality. It will make you feel comfortable.
2. **Keep an eye on your breathing.** When you're at home set aside ten minutes a day to take long, deep breaths. It will help you relax and find a greater connection with yourself.
3. Take **videos with your phone**. It may sound silly, but the

first exercise I teach my students is just that. Recording fictitious conversations, perhaps half or full-length and then watching yourself again is a useful observation exercise that will allow you to see where you can improve.

4. **Speak slower than usual**. Again, this may seem like an odd exercise, but people with charisma convey calmness with their words. Very often people speak too quickly and this conveys some anxiety or otherwise agitation. Practice this at home by speaking in slow motion and articulating syllables very slowly for 15 minutes a day. When you are with others slow down your speaking if you notice that you are agitated.

5. **Look in the mirror naked 10 minutes a day.** I learned this trick from Oliviero Toscani, the famous photographer. Looking at ourselves naked increases our self-awareness. Isn't it amazing?

6. **Give yourself small daily challenges.** Asking a waiter for advice, talking to a bartender or helping a stranger can help you step out of your comfort zone.

7. **Firm handshake, always**. Non-verbal language is so powerful. Always be assertive when interfacing physically. Hugs, handshakes and pats on the back should be vigorous.

8. **Open up**. Don't keep an attitude of closure. Learn to let your body, especially your upper body (shoulders, torso, pelvis) communicate a sense of openness instead of closure.

9. **Try not to procrastinate**. When you are faced with a decision, even a small one, express your opinion clearly and decisively. Yes or no. This is a powerful indicator of personality.

10. **When you panic, listen**. An old trick that always works.

If you're feeling overwhelmed by your emotions get the other person to talk, perhaps by asking them questions. You'll take your time, calm down, and the other person will be satisfied with your curiosity.

11. **Ask lots of questions.** As with the previous tip, asking lots of questions allows you to get to know the other person better, satisfy their desire to talk (everyone loves to talk about themselves) and better organize the conversation.

12. **Talk less about yourself.** Try not to make monologues about yourself. People with charisma focus on the other person and not just themselves.

13. **Learn relational storytelling.** Convey your values through your personal stories, anecdotes and tales. It's the best way to engage our interlocutor and at the same time tell something about ourselves. I often talk about it in my podcast.

14. **When you can, sing**. That's right. Singing and dancing (even in the shower!) help you get unstuck and let go. Make this technique part of your routine.

15. **Bring the discussion to "your" topics.** As soon as you can, try to get the other person to talk about topics close to you. You will feel more inspired and the conversation will be more engaging.

16. **Get carried away**. Don't be too brainy, don't think about what you have to say, and don't be too mentally hyperactive. Try to relax, listen actively and contribute quality topics to the conversation.

17. **Verbalize your discomfort.** This trick is used by many speakers at the beginning of a presentation. Phrases such as *"I feel a bit tense" put the* speaker in a state of connection with you. Don't be ashamed to say it - only a strong person

can demonstrate that!

18. **You're kidding**. That's right. At those times we are very nervous and because of that we become "awkward". Joking about the fact that you're not the best communicator in the world will help relieve the tension and lighten you up.

19. **Tap into your sensitive side**. If you consider yourself a sensitive person, you have a plus that can resonate with many people. Don't be ashamed to say it, see it as a plus that can connect you more authentically with others.

20. **Read a lot, every day.** Reading allows you to have new topics of discussion all the time, as well as gaining a richer vocabulary and a more complete view of the world.

21. **Think that you're not doing anything wrong.** Whether it's a cold approach or a chat between colleagues, remember that you don't want to eat anyone, you simply want to communicate, which is the most human and natural thing there is.

22. **Remember that your limitations are not seen by others.** Your interlocutors don't have a magic mirror and can't read your mind, believe me. Probably no one thinks you're "clumsy", it's your own thought and is likely to be limiting.

23. **Just be yourself.** We can't always win. Some people are good at some things, others at others. I'm sure you've got some good qualities too: don't keep them hidden!

7

Why do people talk even when they don't know the topic being talked about?

People talk even when they don't know the subject matter because of **fear of judgment** and underlying **insecurity.**

In my experience I have noticed how **all confident people have the humility to admit their "ignorance on the subject".**

Only a strong and decisive person is in fact able to verbalize a weakness.

People who are insecure and afraid of judgement, on the other hand, find it easier to talk to hide their fears.

There is also a kind of **confirmation bias**, whereby **if we start to talk about a topic we have to confirm this knowledge of ours** precisely to avoid an embarrassment.

I explain this with an intuitive example: as soon as we tell a **lie**, since we cannot go back, all our statements will go to confirm that lie.

People may therefore talk to **hide their frailties** or **fear** of **judgement**.

But we must not forget that many do so because, in their hearts, they are convinced that they are competent.

Ignorant people, by definition, ignore.

They also ignore that they are ignorant, and with that the circle closes.

8

LOVE AND RELATIONSHIPS

9

What can we do to limit misunderstandings in relationships?

There is something we can do to limit misunderstandings which, by their nature, are inevitable.

We can try to think before we speak, to find the right words to limit misunderstanding. We can define, before enunciating, the emotional goal we wish to affect.

Choose the right themes, the right vocabulary, the right metaphors.

If nothing else, we'll have a clear rationalized (and emotionalized) idea of what we mean.

In this way I cannot say that misunderstandings will disappear. I can say, however, that the number and intensity of misunderstandings will decrease.

That's the trick: stop, think about the what, the how, and with what weighty words to express our thoughts.

What emotion we want to visit.

It's not easy, it takes a lot of practice.

There are also some blocking factors: the social environment, for example. And feelings like anger, shame and shyness.

But the moment we can block the instinct to re-process the thought, the quality of communication will increase considerably. And improving communication will improve our relationships. And by extension our lives.

10

How to get over unrequited love?

I know how it feels, and I also know that it **is possible to get out of it by limiting the damage**.

Unrequited love is always a tough nut to crack. As a relationship communication coach, I think I can give you some helpful tips for dealing with this difficult time in your life.

Here's my contribution.

- **Recalibrate your emotional compass.** Have it pointed at you, not the other person. I know it's hard, but it's the starting point to begin the new journey. You have to take charge of your life again, and that takes a huge initial commitment, like any habit. As the days go by it will become easier and easier.
- **No contact.** Brutal technique, but it works. Don't put the knife in, because every message you send will plunge you into oblivion. Cut off contact with him/her for at least a couple of weeks. It will help you see things more clearly.
- **Find sweet distractions.** They'll help you take your mind

off things. Go out, experience things, get back in touch with your old friends. Occupy your time and avoid being alone and isolating yourself from the world. Wallowing in your grief will get you nowhere.

- **If you must cry, cry.** Cry with all your heart, express all your pain. It's the most natural thing there is, and it helps you feel better.
- **Only talk to people who have lived it.** Many people will try to give you unsolicited advice. They are your friends, and they want to help you but don't realize that they often do only harm. Listening to them all will create enormous confusion in you. Give yourself limits, and listen only to the opinions of those who have experienced a similar situation to yours. Remember that advice is a form of nostalgia!
- **Think about timing.** Often in life the time factor is crucial. And we can't control it. It happens to fall in love with a person who at that moment doesn't want to commit, perhaps because they have just broken up. We can't intervene on this, and speeding up the timing wouldn't help anyone, on the contrary, it would fuel confusion on an emotional level.
- **Don't ask yourself why.** There are some things you can't control. Every person is unique, they have their own life, values and feelings. If love is unrequited it doesn't mean you haven't done enough, it just means you are looking for gold where there is no gold. You can keep digging, but you'll only find stones of little value.
- **Abandon the will to control.** See above.
- **Are you idealizing it?** Ask yourself if you are in love with the person or with the idea of being with that person. If the love is not reciprocated there are good chances that your

brain really loves the idea of spending time with someone who doesn't want you, but these are just images more like daydreams than real ambitions.

- **You can't force anyone to love you.** This is the most brutal truth of all. Feeling bad about unrequited love is natural. We mentally project ourselves into a rosy future with the other person, and this expectation is disappointed. It's very painful, I know, but obviously that wasn't the right person at the right time.

- **Don't exaggerate.** Everything will seem insurmountable now. Be concrete and realistic, and give things the right weight. Don't exaggerate.

- **In a few years you'll look back on this.** And you'll smile. Believe me. What you're experiencing today is an emotional whirlwind that seems to have no exit. Tomorrow you'll evaluate it more carefully and with hindsight you'll classify it as a very normal and nostalgic "crush".

11

If a girl writes to a guy all day, does that mean she's in love?

I express my opinion as a communication coach. While each case requires a more in-depth analysis, I can say offhand that writing to a guy all day long **is never a sign of love**.

I see this behavior more as

1. a **continuous search for attention and confirmation, a** symptom of fragility and insecurity
2. as a passive-aggressive **attempt to control** the other…

I repeat: every relationship is its own story, but here I think **we are confusing the word love** with the word "**obsession**".

This kind of behavior is not healthy. Sure, when we are infatuated with someone there is a risk of "losing our jug", but I can say with reasonable certainty that **love does not involve constant demands for attention or control** over the other.

Some time ago a guy in his thirties contacted me for a course to improve his communication in the relational field. Everything went well and after a few sessions he started dating a new girl. He liked her and was curious to get to know her better.

Too bad this woman began to shower him from the first weeks with "love" messages at all hours of the day and night.

My pupil was frightened, and asked my advice.

I told him that love is about writing a message when we have **something special** to say, chalking up words and emotions to deliver them to our partner at the right time. Love is above all **EQUILIBRIUM** that is created between two people.

These **compulsive attitudes** in the vast majority of cases are the antechamber of a strong quarrel, or in any case a symptom of something wrong, of a gear that does not do its job.

Love is **RESPECT** for individual freedom. If we want to control the other we are failing this founding principle, so no, **it is not love but obsession**.

Something quite different and extremely dangerous.

12

The girl I have a crush on says she likes me but won't commit to a relationship. What do I do?

I'm anticipating right now that what I'm going to say is going to hurt you.

Let's start with an assumption: these situations are quite common.

Many of my students have been faced with this Unknown and my suggestion has always been the same: **let it go**.

I know it's gonna hurt, I know you're gonna cry.

But what if I told you that the only REAL card you can play is this one?

You can't force someone to change their mind with logic, much less about something as valuable as relationships.

In your case, I understand you have a crush on her. This is a very powerful indicator that goes to confirm what I was thinking, which is that there is a **huge emotional imbalance between you and her.**

What does this mean?

Simply put, **the emotional investment you can guarantee her is far greater than what she can guarantee you**.

And that's not good, because in relationships you need an **emotional balance** distributed equally among the parties involved.

Remember how I told you earlier that letting her go is the only strategy that can give you a chance?

I'll try to explain why.

If you keep running after her in this state of infatuation, **you will** simply **push her away even more**.

We are strange beings, we humans.

We find almost disreputable what we can have with ease and absolutely intriguing what we cannot have.

Only by detaching yourself from her, living your life, grinding out experiences will you be able to generate an **emotional reset**, to **make yourself see with new eyes**.

And this process takes time.

At the moment as mentioned **the emotional investment is unbalanced**.

I don't rule out that if you can handle the situation "like a man" by accepting her choice and putting the **focus on yourself** more than her there might be a rethink.

Timing is everything in life, and if she is your soulmate you will see that in some bizarre way your paths will meet again.

13

How can I "destroy" an idealized love?

We've all been there. It hurts. And I must say, **it's not easy to remove from our minds** that idea that goes by the name of "what if…"

When we talk about **"idealized" love** we refer to that condition in which the imaginative part inexorably overpowers the realistic part. This allows us to **live a real daydream** that overwhelms us emotionally and sometimes torments us.

To idealize a person is to elevate them to semi-god status, and this is always a very dangerous process.

As mentioned, at first one idealizes the partner, exalting his merits and remaining blind to any imperfection.

After that, our brains begin to fantasize to the extreme, polarizing emotions toward a totalizing outcome where the relationship is, literally, **perfect**.

Now, this perfection is only **apparent**, and is the result of the multiplication between the desire to obtain (or maintain) love and the idealistic drive of our being, often and willingly influenced by movies and literature.

In reality, idealized love does not exist.

What exists is love for the idea of being in love.

That's right.

You're not in love. You're enraptured by the idea of being in love.

You like the idea. You fantasize, put it on a pedestal. But it's just a mental film.

That's how it works in most cases.

<h1 style="text-align:center">14</h1>

How to manage a relationship with a colleague?

I'll give you one piece of dispassionate advice: **never start a relationship with a colleague**.

Really, don't.

I haven't experienced it myself, but **a good friend of mine** has been together for a couple of years with a co-worker. They work in a store: he's the manager, she's a salesperson.

If in the first few weeks the **mystery and taste of the forbidden** can make the clandestine relationship exciting, after a few months you'll find that it isn't anymore.

Everything turns into a **routine** in which free time and work mix until the whole relationship deteriorates.

The reasons are really simple, and the last one will put you off:

1. It's gonna be hard to **keep the others in the dark about** this.
2. Your coworkers are gonna start **gossiping**
3. You can no longer be completely **yourself** when you're in the office.
4. Many **companies** do not accept relationships between colleagues
5. **Embarrassing** moments will multiply
6. You always meet in a completely unsuitable **context**
7. See you around. **Always**.
8. Work will enter your **love life,** and it will never leave.
9. What about the **holidays**? How would you do it?

I told you there's one last reason, much more vicious than the others.

There you go.

If the couple breaks up, **you'll be forced to see their ugly face, every day,** until one of them changes jobs. It could be years.

Think it through.

15

What to do if you are in love with a girl, but haven't opened up to her for many years?

Let's start with a simple and **brutal** assumption: she after so many years has an image of you that most likely does **NOT match that of** a potential **partner**.

This is coming from a guy who was engaged for 7 years to her best friend!

There are 2 ways you can follow (one immediate and devastating and one slow but potentially effective)

1. **You make a romantic declaration.** Argh! This is what any man with no experience in this area would do, generating embarrassment and making the situation worse. Of course, love could also be reciprocated but according to my experience as a coach in this area I can assure you that it happens one time in a million. Doing

this **will hardly get you the desired result**.

2. **You work on yourself to change the image she has of you**. That's right. We said she's used to having a certain kind of relationship with you. She sees you as a **friend**. You need to change the image she projects of you, and to do that sometimes you need to **detach in** stages. Start dating other girls, get passionate about new things, work on your physique and your life goals. Most importantly, start taking a **little something out of** your relationship. You got that right, take a little something out of it.

You have to make her understand that **you are the center of the world now**, not her.

Both **physical** and **psychological detachment is** necessary to achieve a rapprochement in the future.

This process takes time, a long time but it is the only opportunity you have to make sure that your love can be reciprocated **after years of friendship**.

16

What does it mean if someone who loves you ignores you and won't tell you why?

First of all I would distinguish the level of "deepening" of the relationship. Speaking of love, we can assume that it is **not something superficial** and long lasting.

In my experience as a communication coach, given these circumstances, I think we can talk about a **passive-aggressive attitude**.

We are derived from primates and one of the primary emotions that governs us is **fear**. And the consequence of fear can manifest in two ways: **flight** or **attack.**

Even on a psychic level we often deal with discomfort either through **silence** or **anger**.

The basis of any loving relationship should be **authentic**

and sincere communication. These kinds of attitudes are **evidence** of the (communicative) **cracks** that exist in the relationship.

Going back to the talk of flight and attack, your partner probably feels he is protecting his own emotional safety by running away from the problem rather than confronting it.

I'm sure he's doing it for the good of the couple but he should realize that by doing so he's destroying the relationship of trust that was previously established.

To remedy the situation I will try to give you some advice

1. **Try talking to him.** Asking calmly what you can do to alleviate this discomfort of his shows your willingness to empathize with him.
2. **Don't put too much weight on his reaction.** He's probably always been like this, you're not going to change that.
3. **Tell him you know this attitude is "protective".** We all have weaknesses and it's not always easy to admit them. Talk to him about your own ways of protecting yourself, perhaps particular ones.
4. **Don't play out disaster scenarios.** No threats, no repercussions, no consequences. Walk in his shoes, try to put yourself in his shoes.

Having said that, however, one big issue remains: **you have a communication problem**. The fact that he says he loves you and then acts this way means there is some "submerged" between you.

Improving communication can transform your relationships, and transforming your relationships improves your life.

What's one "man problem" that women wouldn't understand?

That many, many men have an **emotional and sensitive side** and that hiding it makes them suffer more than you can imagine.

And that no, **we're not always strong**.

One of the most argued issues by my students is just that.

"What will women think if I show my emotional side or weaknesses?"

In contemporary society there is still a very strong stigma in relation to the combination of man and emotion.

Man must be confident, brave, fearless. Yet most male beings do not feel this way. We are **forced into a role** that fits us tightly and fails to fully represent our nuances and character.

The biggest "guy" problem that women wouldn't understand is

that we hide because **we fear their judgment**.

We all have our insecurities, it's just that in order to avoid disappointing female expectations we wear masks that fit tightly.

BEING SENSITIVE MEN ISN'T A BAD THING.

In fact, it can be a plus.

As I always explain to all my students, **sensitivity** can be an **incredible advantage** in winning and maintaining a relationship. It is a **differentiating element** that can make us stand out within the group.

In a world populated by *"fake alphas"* (they feel like it, but women understand it's a "cover") who flaunt confidence and lack of feelings (the so-called "stro**i") the man who admits to having some weak points stands out for sincerity.

He can **empathize more with women**, who tend to be emotional beings. He can find new, unprecedented, unexpected points of contact for women.

I always say that the true *alpha* man is the one who is able to admit that he is NOT an *alpha*, and doesn't even want to be one.
   What could be more alpha than a man who can admit he's not an alpha?
   Only those with great self-awareness are able to do this!
   We're no longer chimps ruling the jungle, contemporary society is complex and **using our sensibilities to our advantage**

may seem like a crazy enough idea to work.

This is confirmed by the **dozens of growth paths that** I have taken with my students who, in fact, have begun to **recognize** and **accept** their sensitive side, greatly improving the quality of their relationships.

If you're interested I talk about this a lot on my podcast.

18

FIRST DATE

<h1 style="text-align:center">19</h1>

What do you think would be the ideal place for a first date?

There are some ideal features for the **perfect place** to take your he or she for the first time. I'm going to describe them now, but first it's best that you know some **guidelines**.

1. **It needs to be a place where conversation is possible.** If the disco is a bad idea, the cinema is a very beginner's choice. Find a place where the music isn't loud and it's comfortable to talk.
2. **No crowded places.** Too many people creates disruption and annihilates intimacy. Look for a nice little place that you know is well attended and never full as an egg.
3. **In that case, better make a reservation.** Always call the bar in the morning (or the night before) to make sure it's open (most pubs close on Mondays, for example) and book a table for two at a certain time. If you can go to book in person even better: you can choose the table that looks best to you (no one likes to sit next to the toilet).
4. **No isolated places.** Having people around puts your

partner at ease, especially for a first date. It can provide a sense of security for both of you. So no horror movie alleys or parking lots, for goodness sake!

5. **No romantic restaurant.** Too busy for a first date. Remember that a first date is an opportunity to get to know and "smell" each other. Inviting your partner to an expensive place would create a lot of awkwardness.

6. **No extreme experiences**. Escape rooms, carnivals, etc. Forget it. The focus needs to be on your conversation, and these are far too demanding activities.

7. **No coffee shop downstairs.** While this is the least worst case scenario, you should try to make this first date something special. It's not nice to find out that your apartment is only 10 meters away from the bar you invited her to.

8. **Favor places you've been to before.** Reviews on Yelp or TripAdvisor can be misleading, as can photos of the place or the service. It's better to go for sure. And when in doubt, if you really want to take her somewhere new, pop in a few days beforehand.

9. **Offer to pay for the drink or the drink.** Be a gentleman, always. If the girl insists, offer to buy her a second round.

But you want to know the perfect place for a first date, right?

The best place to take a girl on a first date is not a place, but a **walk**.

That's right: propose that you meet her somewhere in the city and go for **a walk together**. You'll stop for a drink as soon as you come across a place that inspires you both, and in the meantime you'll have **already started to get to know each other** (and released the accumulated tension).

Opting for the walk will allow you to not go crazy looking for the perfect venue and you can find a place that definitely "inspires" both of you. There is therefore also a sense of discovery that can come together.

The choice of *"what we WANT"* is already a nice icebreaker that, in between streets, will allow you to learn more about your partner's tastes.

And if the venue turns out to be a package deal, no harm done: *misery loves company.* Next!

I can tell you from experience: there's nothing more **nerve-wracking than** waiting for a date in a club… The idea of a walk really lightens the atmosphere and you can decide together how to continue the evening.

And remember: you know what the goal of a first date is?

Get a second one, of course!

20

How not to look "desperate" on a first date

Not looking "desperate" on the first date (and the second, and the third…) is a real necessity for many males out there.

I offer you **five tips** to help you be at your **best** with your partner:

1. **Ask yourself if you're desperate.** I am. The first step is to ask yourself if you are really that desperate. You are probably referring to the fact that first dates are rather rare events in your life and therefore load this event with tension. This very tension will make you feel needy. Trust me. Try to live it as an experience, thinking that there will be other occasions. And remember: *if it goes wrong, remember that she judged your way of communicating, not you as a person.* So you can sleep soundly without blaming yourself too much.

2. **Easy with the compliments.** Politeness is fine, but don't go overboard with compliments. And remember: girls get

thousands of compliments for their bodies (cf. "You have *beautiful eyes*" and "*you have a beautiful smile*") but definitely less for their intelligence (which is much more remarkable). Listen to her carefully, and if you do, compliment her on her ideas and brains. She will immediately notice the difference between you and the usual guys.

3. **Create a little mystery.** Repeat with me, "*I'm not going to tell her everything right away, I'm going to leave a little mystery.*" You got it? Good, you're well on your way. I know that when we are caught up in the enthusiasm we have the tendency to answer like a machine gun to every question, but please try to answer in an evasive way, at least sometimes. It will generate more interest, and therefore more questions. It will benefit the dialogue.

4. **Don't flaunt.** Don't flaunt the confidence you don't have, don't flaunt the wealth you don't have, don't flaunt things you don't know. Because exaggeration never pays off, and it is well known that those who only talk about themselves in this way hide enormous fragility and low self-esteem.

5. **She's flawed too.** I don't want to be too brutal, but often a lot of guys idealize the partner with whom they have to meet and then make horrible mistakes. It's time to remove that veil of magic from the girl's head and start thinking that she's a person like all the others. Yes, they do it too and yes, even they just woke up can have a breath that makes welding.

21

How to impress a girl on a first date?

This is a **good list of things to do to impress a girl** on a first date. The last one always works

- **It shows you're capable of making decisions.** That's right. You have to have a pulse when it comes to deciding where to go, what to do, how to proceed with the evening. And do it by always being polite and with the utmost respect for the person in front of you. Women don't like people who are *lame* even when it comes to deciding where to dine.
- **Talk about yourself, but through stories.** Rather than giving a sermon about how handsome you are and how good you are, learn how to tell about yourself through storytelling. Your anecdotes will tell a lot about who you are, the challenges you've faced and the plans you have for the future. With the plus of not boring you.
- **No frills, it's practicality**. Don't try to impress with big cars, expensive restaurants or grand gestures. It's no use. That's all appearance: what's the point?
- **Manage your body language well.** If you learn to do this

you will be able to impress her without uttering a single word. You'll send very powerful non-verbal messages that tell a lot about you.

- **Admit your weaknesses.** This is an attitude that not everyone has the courage to have. Are you sensitive? Say it! Do you get emotional watching Bambi? Say it! Only a real man is comfortable communicating his weaknesses. Most men aim to hide and mystify them.
- **Be self-deprecating:** see above
- **Go out of your way to make her feel comfortable.** This will facilitate the whole conversation.
- **Make her laugh.** But with intelligence. No movie-star jokes!

I told you about a tip that always works. Here we go.

- **Listen to her**. That's right. Simple, right? Not quite. We often get carried away by our emotions and want the spotlight to be on us. It's natural, but it doesn't lead to great results. If you show that you actively listen, you'll be different from 99% of the men she's met before. Ask her questions, ask her to elaborate on a topic, rephrase concepts and show that you understand. Everyone loves to be heard.

22

What not to do on a first date?

I think I can give you some advice (unisex of course).

- **Don't get your hopes up.** You are not a robot and cannot control each other. Simply live the experience enjoying the surprises this event will bring.
- **Don't force things.** If they're going to happen, they're going to happen.
- **Don't talk about sex.** Or politics. Nor religion or "hot" topics. It's best to wait a while: after all, it's just a first meeting, right?
- **Don't bring gifts.** There is not yet the confidence necessary for such a gesture.
- **Don't just talk about your problems.** You can talk about them, sure, but discreetly. The concept is very simple: time is short and the opportunity is unique. Why negate such a beautiful opportunity?
- **Don't reach for your hands.** I don't have to explain this one to you, do I?
- **Don't be late.** Ten minutes is okay, an hour is definitely

not. And just in case, always let them know in good time that you've had a setback so the other person can make arrangements.

- Don't **EVER talk about your exes**. Seriously, don't. And if the other person does, I have a phrase for you that you can reuse if necessary.
- *"We're short on time, and I have a lot of questions to ask you to get to know you better, since you interest me. Let's not waste it talking about the past!"*
- **Don't lie.** We all have weaknesses. When a lie, big or small, is about to start, stop it immediately. Otherwise you will pay the consequences sooner or later.
- **Don't be disinterested.** If you've been taught that being a jerk is part of the seduction process, you may be missing a piece. When you have a person in front of you, you should always show sincere interest in their arguments. To be mysterious, there are other shores and other more suitable situations.
- **Don't kiss him on the doorstep at the end of the night.** That only works in the movies. Do it when you're in your ascending phase.
- **Don't mince words.** An "I love you" on the first date can derail any good intention. Ted Mosby's word.
- **Don't overdo it.** Don't try to impress her with special effects. A walk is fine.

23

What to say to a girl after a first date?

Here's a **set of tips (the last one is key)** I feel like giving you on what to say to a girl after the first date (assuming **it went well**).

- **Don't ask "how did I do? "**. For heaven's sake. You need to be able to tell with reasonable certainty whether the meeting went well or not. Ditto with the very banal *"did you have a good time?"*.
- **It creates emotional tension.** We're all a bit of dreamers, we like to fantasize. If the first date went properly, let some time pass before you contact her again (even a couple of days!).
- **Don't be in a hurry to text her**. A little mystery, come on. Let her fantasize a little. A sweet expectation never killed anyone.
- **Don't do anything that identifies you as "needy"**. Calmness is the virtue of the strong. If you self-talk the

consequences will be devastating.

- **It brings attention to pleasant memories.** When you reconnect it brings back the brightest moments of the evening. They're a great hook.
- **It shows he listened to her.** Pull that detail out of your hat that she thought had gone unnoticed. You'll impress her.
- **What about the second date?** Don't make the mistake of waiting too long to ask for a second date. Do it already during the first one if you notice that you are in the right "flow".

And if you're waiting for the last piece of advice, **the most important one**, here we are.

- **After the first date, if she is really interested, she will write to you.** If this happens to you, consider yourself lucky: that girl really cares about you!

24

What should you know before you kiss someone?

- **You have to create an emotional "escalation".** For this you have to be good at involving the partner with gestures and words. It must be born that flame that grows and grows. The kiss will then come by itself.
- **The kiss, believe it or not, is prepared "before".** That's right, you have to do a good job of suggesting emotions BEFORE you go out, in the days leading up to it. Create an expectation, scenarios together, get her/him excited and wanting that kiss.
- **Never kiss "cold."** Kissing is the end point of a journey of getting to know each other. You have to create physical tension before approaching such an intimate gesture. And trust me: the girl will make it very clear to you whether or not you should kiss her.
- **Don't wait to drive her home to do it.** Bad idea, beginner's idea. You need to clearly understand that the time to try is when you are in the *ascending phase*. At the

end of the night the emotional parabola is *downward*. Much better sooner than later, believe me: the evening will take a turn for the better.

- **Don't verbalize your desire to kiss her.** *"Sorry, can I kiss you?"* No, thank you. Or even *"I really want to kiss you."* like the famous slogan says, just do it.
- **It's all about timing.** 99% of dates fail because you don't act with the right method and with the right timing. If a girl goes out with you she shows that she has an interest, don't ruin it with your haste or your shyness!

25

Does there have to be physical contact on the first date?

The answer to your question is: **YES, you need to have one or more physical contacts with the girl even (and especially) on the first date.**

Let's make a small premise: we're not talking about erotic touches but light touches that make sense.

We all hate being touched when not requested, and the risk of appearing inappropriate is always just around the corner.

Physical contact is crucial when getting to know each other, we cannot overlook perhaps the most important of the five senses.

The mistake that many guys make is precisely this: to think of being **inappropriate** and keep their partner at a distance as if they were about to commit something unacceptable. Or the exact opposite, that is to say being **harassed**.

The good news is this: if the girl + there with you to some extent feels a curiosity about you. It means that you have worked well before and have managed to **establish even a minimal relationship of trust**.

And it is for this very reason that **this trust must NEVER be betrayed**. It takes delicacy. You have to know how to do it, don't improvise.

When in doubt, don't touch, you risk damage!

Unfortunately, many of my students have no half measures: either **they "extend themselves"** too much or **they don't even contemplate a touch**.

Body language is an art that must be learned and practiced with a lot of dedication.

What I can recommend is

1. Always put the person in front of you at ease
2. Try to touch, for example, his hand while you are walking together. If he withdraws you will immediately understand that you have to stop and that this is not a good time.
3. If the first tactile signals give a positive feedback, you can start an escalation that will lead to a kiss.

The first acquaintance relationship between humans happens just as it does in the animal world. There is a visual first impression, an olfactory first impression, an auditory first

impression (your voice and tone) and yes, even a **tactile first impression**.

If you have not created the slightest physical contact, it will be practically impossible to achieve a kiss (sense of taste).

Through touches, hand games and complicit smiles, an understanding is created. Yes, that very understanding: sexual.

One last piece of advice, don't wait to drive her home to kiss her. It's absolutely the wrong time to do it. Trust me!

26

BETTER CONVERSATIONS

<h1 style="text-align:center">27</h1>

What does a good conversation consist of?

Imagine a **good conversation** as a **classical symphony**, where dozens of instruments take turns creating different melodies.

In order to define a "good" conversation here are the **parameters I consider fundamental:**

1. The **time** dedicated to each interlocutor
2. The **commonality of** topics and communicative objectives
3. Openness to **new ideas**
4. Authentic **listening** and **respect for** others

Here are additional characteristics that I believe are crucial to a **good conversation.**

- **Reciprocity**. The topics are of sincere interest to both. The passion is mutual and there are obvious elements of contact.

- **Emotionality.** A good conversation never leaves you cold. It can overwhelm you and make you experience emotions. From laughter to sadness.
- **Authentic listening.** One listens to the other attentively, without thinking about the answer to give but focusing on the other's words. Body language also communicates attention and predisposition toward the other.
- **No distractions.** In a good conversation there should be no distracting elements. So no cell phone in hand or eyes in the air.
- **Stories.** Stories are a very powerful way to convey personal values and goals. They are hardly boring and can tell a lot about us.
- **Memorable details and descriptions.** The ability to bring our story to life for the other person through excellent use of vocabulary and adjectives.
- **Appropriate body language**. It is used to support words.
- **Communicative calm.** And tone of voice and pace appropriate to the context.
- **No interrogation.** No barrage of one-way questions. Much better the indirect questions that smell less of inquisition.
- **Emotional attunement**. To put it another way: empathy. Really feeling what the other person is feeling.
- **Involving everyone.** If there are more than two people, never leave anyone out of the conversation. Everyone needs to be involved.
- **Fairness of timing.** In a good conversation A talks as much as B. No one monopolizes the conversation but there is equity in time management.
- **Equity of Investment.** Emotional investment should also

be high and divided equally between the parties.

- **Mystery.** Speeches that leave a veil of mystery are certainly more intriguing than completely logical ones.
- **Use of poetic/metaphorical language.** Logical and rational discourse should still make use of rhetorical figures such as metaphors and similes.
- **Using pauses.** Pauses are the punctuation of the voice. If well used
- **Few pleasantries.** Leave the pleasantries at the beginning and then move on to more concrete things.

28

What is the best way to start an online conversation?

Think about it: an online conversation is nothing more than the **digital transposition of** a normal conversation in **real life**.

The fact that it is done through a computer in no way precludes the presence of all those elements that we normally consider.

Here are some examples

1. **Context**. You need to understand what the context is in which you are moving. Where are you located? On a dating app? On a sewing forum? On WhatsApp with a colleague? Try to understand what the purpose of your communication is, adapted to the medium you are using.
2. **The motivation to approach.** Why are you approaching? Why do you want to converse? Even in real life we have different communication goals. You might start chatting to ask for advice, schoolwork or to ask for information.

Just like it happens on the street or otherwise in real life.

3. **The Degree of Confidence.** This is the most important element. How well do you know this person? Is this a "cold" approach or do you already know each other? In the case of cold approaches I can give you some advice below.

4. **Your "un" stated goals.** Yes, if we ask ourselves this question we may have some goals that we don't want to reveal at first. It's the classic example of asking for a lighter to start a conversation with a pretty girl. Always ask yourself: what do I want to achieve?

There are many "starters" for starting a cold conversation online. What I can tell you is to always be original, polite **and** emotional.

Why do I say "emotional"?

Simple, because in the digital context (e.g. of a dating app) you get so many conversational requests that it's really hard to hit the target.

Personally, I pay a lot of attention to vocabulary.

I always ask myself: what kind of emotion do I wish to "trigger" with this first message of mine?

Do I want to seem nice and a little crazy?

Then I'll write something like, *"Let's get right to the important stuff and skip the pleasantries: who's your favorite Spice Girl?"*

Joking aside, I can't tell you exactly what to write (I'd have to know you, your passions, your way of doing things, etc.) but I can give you one piece of advice: **DON'T BE BANAL.**

Never start with a **compliment about the body, the eyes, the lips**.

Never start with a **hello** or a **hey**.

Don't ever start by peppering her with **questions**.

Never write a **papyrus**.

Always show that you are very observant and focused on a few details that will amaze her.

DISTINGUISH yourself, try to be original, different from everyone else.

Don't just write the first thing that comes to mind. Spend some time because in order to give emotion and differentiate yourself you will need to create a truly unique message.

29

How do you start a conversation?

Every **good conversation** cannot be without one really crucial element: **observation**.

Here's a technique I've tested in my coaching programs to help my learners when they don't know how to start a dialogue.

1. Observe your interlocutor carefully and look for some **useful cues** in their clothing or expression. It can be a wrinkled expression, a pair of ethnic earrings, a particular pair of shoes and whatever else.
2. Next you **ask** an **indirect question**, but also include an **assumption**.
3. Here's an example: "I see you have … I guess you're …."
4. Result: "I see you're wearing ethnic earrings, I guess you're a big fan of travel."

This technique is able to generate **immediate attention** because it involves the interlocutor in the first person, who will feel "called upon". All this without the heaviness of a direct question and demonstrating a spirit of observation, which is appreciated by most people.

30

How can you keep the level of conversation up?

Keeping the level of a conversation "high" is a real art. Here I offer a series of tips to avoid unwanted yawns

- **You always play on emotions.** It's hard to get bored when a story is moving. Make good use of emotional storytelling techniques, which include building suspense and aiming to stir up emotions in the other person. It's mostly about evoking primary emotions, such as fear, surprise or disgust.
- **Be the one to make connections.** Remember that your goal must be to steer the conversation. To do this, you must be an excellent listener, capable of "attacking the button" as soon as the opportunity arises. Every sentence you say can open a thousand doors to as many insights: keep your ears open and try to understand what the other person needs and wants.
- **Generate curiosity.** Try to leave a few windows open, don't reveal everything right away - this will keep the focus on what you're saying.

- **Make the other person immerse themselves in "your" world.** Use detailed descriptions to immerse the other person in your stories. Always start with small details and then describe the environment surrounding your story. Remember to let all five senses speak, and that olfactory memories are among the most powerful. Don't just tell the story, try to "see with words" so the other person doesn't get bored.
- **Ask quality questions.** That's right. Questions have the unique power to ignite our attention. They are great insights as long as they are relevant and unfastened at the right time. Don't be trite. A question like *"how are you?"* doesn't add quality to the dialogue. *"What was the last thing you were excited about"* is better.
- **From time to time, lower the tone of your voice.** The old teacher's trick that always works to keep the students in class quiet.
- **Don't be monotonous**. There's nothing more boring than a person who talks in a machine or keeps the same tone of voice. Try to modulate the way you speak by emphasizing, slowing down and speeding up when appropriate.
- **Give clear verbal commands.** When you want to show that you are in control of the conversation, you can try giving verbal commands (usually in the imperative mode) to better govern the dialogue. E.g. *so tell me what ... / give me a clear example of ... / remind me what that .... was called.*
- **Make assumptions and ask indirect questions.** This technique can also awaken our interlocutor from his sweet torpor, and should be balanced with direct questions. To keep the dialogue from sounding like an interrogation I often use the formula *"I see that ... I imagine that ...".* This

serves to tease the conversation and invigorate the focus.

- **Remember verbalized mirroring.** When the other person speaks, show your interest by occasionally rephrasing the concepts they express. In addition to showing altruism, you will be giving a very clear message: I am listening to you!

- **Manage the "communication ping pong" as best you can.** We all like to talk about ourselves, but we need to have a certain measure in doing so. Conversation is like a game of ping pong: it takes two to play. Keep your antennae straight and always look to see if you're taking up too much communicative space. If you do all the talking, your interlocutor will start thinking about something else. This principle also applies in the opposite case.

- **Repeat the name of the interlocutor.** This is also a powerful and atavistic stimulus to awaken the attention of the person in front of us.

31

What's the best way to get out of a conversation where there's no end in sight?

I'm assuming this is a **boring conversation** (we'll see the heated discussion later). E.g. *Your neighbour has started to attack you about work to be done next year on the gutters.*

The trick, as always, is to **work on your emotions**.

Just so you know:

- Status of the interlocutor A **excited**
- Status of caller B **bored**

To get out of a conversation like this I would use a peremptory

"I really have to run."

or I would announce my departure due to business commitments

"I have to go, I have an appointment in 15 minutes."

The trick is to **shift the focus** from wanting to leave to an **external factor** (*work, appointments, kids, co-worker*).

The more **specific the motivation, the** more effective it will be. In any case, always be very careful to use the **principle of urgency** sparingly.

Compare

- *"I have to go."*
- *"I have to go because I have to be at Maurizio's in twenty minutes because mum isn't well and I have to help him do some renovations around the house."*
- (we've also thrown in the **emotional element** here).

The more emotional the message, the more effective it will be. We now analyze a **second case**:

- Status of the interlocutor A **angry**
- Status of caller B **angry**

If it were two madmen arguing angrily and unable to reach an agreement instead I suggest you use the **most powerful phrase** in such cases:

YOU'RE RIGHT. I'M SORRY. WHAT CAN I DO TO MAKE IT UP TO YOU?

This phrase may be controversial, but it is **technically unassailable**.

As it is **tripartite,** it is also possible to use **only one of the three parts.**

(E.g. *"sorry"*)

or **pair them**

(E.g. *"You're right, what can I do to make it right?"*)

For a **nuclear effect** use the full formula above.

32

How can I improve my public speaking skills?

One piece of advice: learn the art of **emotional storytelling**.

In my experience as a communications trainer, I've found that there's **nothing more persuasive than a well-told story** that touches the emotional chords of your audience.

I often notice that many speakers try to justify their reasoning with logic. They have great difficulty in **transmitting their values** precisely because they do not activate in the audience that part of the brain that governs emotions.

To persuade there are no tricks and gimmicks: you have to be able to make the other person see the world from a new point of view, **without boring them**.

Learning how to tell stories (and put them in the right contexts) will allow you to be persuasive and keep your audience on their toes until the last minute.

33

BREAKING UP AND TAKING BACK

34

I want to break up with my girlfriend. What are the best ways to do that?

Breaking up is always painful, for both of us.

I can give you some advice.

The last one is the most powerful, trust me it doesn't miss a beat.

But first remember:

1. **There is no such thing as the "right time."** Coming up is anniversary, Valentine's Day, summer vacation booked together, Christmas, Easter, Boxing Day, her birthday. Don't waver on "when" to say it. Say it as soon as possible.
2. **Know that no matter how hard you try, it will be terrible.** It's going to suck, because even though you decided to break up with that person you had some good times and you're attached to them.
3. **Make it as "least pitiful" as possible.** No drama, no

screaming, no second thoughts, no goodbyes via What-sApp. Breaking up already sucks, don't make it even more awful and childish.

4. **Try to be clear and honest.** Admit your mistakes, bring attention to yourself and your feelings (you'll soon discover the world's most unequivocal phrase)

5. **Cut the reports. This is a FUNDAMENTAL step.** Do it, at least for a while. Both of you will need a silent pause to grieve. No texting, no missing you. And if she writes you tell her that this will make it worse.

6. **Try to be firm.** Don't hesitate, try to be clear and explain your reasons. She will try to fight you, and if you are not decisive she will somehow manage to make you take a step back (bad idea).

7. **Leave no room for second thoughts.** There's nothing worse than giving false hope.

There is, however, an **UNCONFUTABLE** phrase for leaving a person.

Think very carefully before you say it, because you can never go back.

This phrase is **"I no longer love you."**

35

My boyfriend and I have picked up and broken up several times. How do I know this is a permanent goodbye?

The answer is simpler than you think: **you decide**.

Certain on-and-offs can go on for years, but if I've learned anything in over 25 years of relationships it's that these situations never lead to anything good.

Sooner or later someone will give the final rip, because if these are congenital attitudes of history it is very rare that they will fix themselves.

If this happens it means that something big is not working. A fundamental mechanism is broken.

I suggest you take the reins, give yourself an ultimatum and get into the mindset that it's going to burn a lot in the moment, but in the long run you'll have made the right choice.

36

What does it mean if she likes me a lot but wants to be alone for a while?

There are 3 cases

1. **She likes you, but not enough to commit to you in a relationship**. In this case, there's little you can do about it: her emotions for you are unrequited and there's a big discrepancy at the level of emotional investment. Read under: you like her a lot more than she likes you.
2. **She likes you, she would also like to be in a relationship but she is in a moment of her life where she is really confused**. It often happens after you break up: being alone is the only solution to elaborate the bad previous experience and forcing a person to start a new relationship is a very, very bad idea (I speak from personal experience)
3. **As you might imagine in this case, timing is crucial**. We're often the right people who meet at the wrong time (and there's nothing we can do about it). I suggest you leave her alone for a while (that's what she asked for after

all!) and wait for better times. In the meantime, live your life!

37

Is love there when you miss your partner?

Short answer: **no**. **Missing** someone is something completely **natural**, but **it is** certainly **not the only indicator** of the presence of the feeling we call **love**.

You can't reduce the most precious of feelings to reason.
"I miss him, so I love him/her."

I'll try to explain why with a **list of thoughts**.

1. **Love is a varied set of sensations.** Lack alone as mentioned is not the indicator, but rather ONE indicator.
2. **Sense of Possession**. We often mask our attraction and need to be with someone with an ill-concealed tendency to possess. Where there is possession there can be no love.
3. **Affective dependence**. It is common to confuse love with something darker and more debilitating: emotional dependence. This does not allow us to clearly evaluate

how we feel, as dependent on the other.

4. **Love is also loneliness**. The ability to be alone for short or long periods of time is the prerogative of a healthy relationship and an adult person.

5. **Love should never hurt**. If this lack causes pain, it's an indicator of an unhealthy relationship, or well, a lack of communication between the partners (*why do I feel bad when it's not there? Why don't we talk about it and work it out?*)

6. **Sense of habit**. Just like when you take the toy away from your newborn, this sense of loss could come from the sudden change of something we were used to.

I know, I was **brutal**, but read on.

Notwithstanding, as we said, that the sense of **lack** is not the only indicator of the feeling of **love**, let's try to understand **what** this feeling **may be due to**.

1. **Attachment**. You are fond of his presence, so you miss him.

2. **Role in your life**. An important piece that you'd like to have around. It's a good start. You'll soon see why.

3. **Not need, but pleasure.** Pleasure of being together, pleasure of sharing experiences and daily moments.

4. **Sharing**. That drive that makes you say "I want to do it with him/her" and would make even a boring afternoon on the couch watching Netflix a memorable experience.

5. **Fantasia**. Everyone is pointing out to you: it's clear as day that you're smitten. You start fantasizing, you have little hearts in your eyes and butterflies in your stomach. Your

brain is in overdrive!

6. **Sense of completeness**. Being with him/her makes you feel better than when you are alone.

38

Can true love be at first sight?

Beware of people who say they fell in love at first sight because

"Who falls in love at first sight betrays at every glance."

Love by definition is a **very deep** feeling.

It's that lever that moves the mountains each of us carries inside.

And no, it can't be "at first sight".

What you call "love" needs to be replaced with **other**, far more fitting **terms.**
Infatuation, interest, sympathy, attraction.
But certainly not **LOVE.**

Attraction is that thing that makes you set your eyes on a beautiful seedling in a nursery.
Love manifests itself by watering it every day, nourishing it with light and, indeed, loving it.

In some cases this "seedling" will have to be moved to another pot because it is **growing**. Often these displacements are painful, often generate doubts, but they are nothing more than the metaphorical transposition of the phases of a relationship.

So on balance **"love at first sight" does not exist**. It is a badly formulated phrase and also the result of a culture, especially in cinema, that has often relied on this concept so abstract and unrealistic.

At first glance there is attraction, which is quite another thing.

39

Why do some people when they break up immediately look for another relationship?

Many people when they break off a relationship will (almost) immediately jump into another relationship for a rather simple reason: they **don't know how to be alone**.

In my experience as a trainer I have answered this question quite often.

This is a question that carries **many nuances** that I will try to argue.

What causes a person to immediately seek another relationship?

1. Emotional Dependence
   Some individuals are characterized by an extreme fragility that leads them to seek support and confirmation in others. This imbalance leads to an obsessive search for a partner able

to satisfy the psychic needs of confirmation and fulfilment that they cannot face alone.

2. Inability to deal with situations independently

This is a classic characteristic of those who, although grown up, still behave like "children". The child places himself at the center of the world and is constantly looking for a "mother" to care for and nurture him.

3. Lack of detachment from a childish logic

Many people, trivially, fail to develop the correct detachment first from their parents and then from their partner(s). This is childish logic. Keep in mind that only through detachment is it possible to create an adult self-image.

4. Creating a fake selfie

Entrusting others with the burden of defining who we are is not only easier, but also definitely cheaper on a psychic level. Detaching from the family nucleus and facing situations "as an adult" requires strength, determination and above all pain. A necessary pain, that many "grown up children" tend to avoid, often for the whole life.

5. Spite. Yes, spite. We often throw ourselves into the arms of another person simply to spite our ex. Often we don't realize it, because it happens at an unconscious level. We want to prove our value, to be still attractive on the market, to make her understand what she has lost.

The **bad news** is that 99% of the time she or he doesn't care, and 100% of the time you prove yourself to be a rookie playing fifth grade games.

Ah, it's scientifically proven that the "fling" that follows a major story doesn't work. EVER.

(unless, of course, the time has passed to "absorb and somatize the grief" of the previous separation).

Please note. There's no such thing as a *nail-biter.*

To borrow an old adage:

"the nail crusher fills time, not the void."

Many of you will agree with me. When a relationship breaks up, we can always talk about **failure**. Failure of expectations, of ideas, but above all of **life projects**.

This **generates an emptiness** within us that is difficult to manage, and we often tend to throw ourselves immediately into another relationship so as not to suffer disproportionately. Here again we talk about a psychic self-protection that, alas, **brings no good**.

Tips for dealing with a break-up situation

1. **Spend some time alone**. When a breakup happens, don't jump right into another story. It won't work. Instead, think about where you can improve.
2. **Improve yourself.** Study, be passionate, read. I know it's

hard not to think about what happened but now it's right to invest in yourself.

3. **Never walk alone.** Seek understanding in your circle of friends, go out, make an effort to create new habits.

I want to give you one last tip.

Never retrace your steps. This advice is brutal but it almost always works. If it helps, think about the fact that in life one **crucial variable** we have no control over is **time**. You were probably the right partner for that person, you just arrived at the wrong time. In many cases it does.

40

OVERCOMING THE FEAR OF TALKING TO PEOPLE

41

I'm a boring person, how can I change?

You are not boring. You **are** simply **not able to best communicate yourself to the world, enhancing yourself through your stories**.

Everyone possesses some specialness. Anyone who has a life, has been a child, and has had a modicum of social interaction has one or more **STORIES** to tell. The point is to **learn how to do it**.

Because let's remember that when we define ourselves as "boring" it trivially means that we are not able to **make ourselves interesting in the eyes of others**, to **engage** and **excite them with our** stories, our words or our experiences.

The good news is that EVERYONE IS SPECIAL and EVERYONE CAN BE INTERESTING.

You don't believe it?

I have a friend who works in a fashion store. Certainly not the most exciting job in the world, is it? Yet she has an **uncanny ability to tell and describe her customers** that leaves me speechless every time.

He knows how to tell his (boring) world impeccably and emotionally.

Have you noticed how there are some people who, as soon as they open their mouths, silence falls and everyone is there with tense ears, even if they are telling about their **trivial day at school**?

What is it about these people that is different from others that draws all the attention to themselves?

It's very simple: they **know how to tell themselves and their stories well, no matter how banal they may be.**

Because at the end of the day, nothing is trivial to others if we can engage them. What is probably missing in your communication is the **ability to emote**.

To summarize: you don't lack topics (unless you've been living in a cryogenic cell your whole life), you don't lack experience. What you lack is the ability to **convey emotion through your experience**.

<h1 style="text-align:center">42</h1>

How to deal with people who only talk about themselves?

For dealing with people who only talk about themselves there is a **very simple** but equally effective **technique.** I teach it to my students that I follow in coaching and I have called it "**the lightning bolt technique**".

It's not what I would call an orthodox technique, but it works.

Let's take a step back first, though.

Why should someone, in a communicative act, not leave space for the interlocutor? Why does he want all the attention on himself? Why doesn't he/she leave room for criticism and comments from the other?

The answer is very simple: **insecurity**.

Focusing on the self has the ultimate goal of repeatedly showing our merits in order to **deflect the attention of our flaws** and **fears**.

Ah, you will tell me, but there are people who talk about themselves in a negative form, simply put **they complain all the time**.

Also for this kind of people I suggest a technique, this one **I called "sly mirroring technique"**.

People who complain all the time as well as those who strut have in common the **characteristic of narcissism** (not the pathological one, the softer one). In essence they are **constantly seeking attention**.

In the first case due to a lack of **self-esteem** and in the second case due to a search for **confirmation**.

What, then, is the "lightning bolt" technique **so effective in dealing with people who only talk about themselves?**

I will be brutal, but in these cases it is necessary to **communicate explicitly what is happening.**

Usually, in the middle of the conversation, I'll **verbalize** something along the lines of, "Did *you know that some scientific research has shown that people who talk about themselves too much are hiding a very pronounced side of insecurity?"*

Or alternatively, *"You know that if you keep talking only about you, leaving no room for other people's opinions and stories, you're showing that you're afraid of judgment?"*

I realize that these phrases are **brutal**, but I assure you that they work precisely because they **put the person in front of a reality that is difficult to refute.**

On the other hand, if you are dealing with **people who complain all the time,** use the **technique of "sly mirroring".**

The purpose is to **exaggerate the complaint to the point where it is** almost comical.

Use it sparingly and only when the complaints are blatantly a search for confirmation bias.

If the interlocutor keeps complaining about the affair with his girlfriend give him what he wants: **confirmation.**

But in doing so **you take** it **to extremes.**

Verbalize using his own words.

If he says that *"it's not like it was in the beginning"* leverage it by saying that you've noticed it too, that all stories are terrible and that you just can't understand how it's possible for him to tolerate this situation. But **do it while smiling under your moustache** (this detail is very important!).

By exaggerating the confirmation bias **you will put the interlocutor in front of the nonsense that he himself is verbalizing until he reflects** on the specific weight of his statements which, in his view, are strong and heavy but which in reality are simple complaints, often without any weight and thrown in just to feel pitied.

Increase the load, exaggerate, mirror **him, give him what he wants until what he says seems ridiculous,** it always works and you will notice that as soon as he realizes the nonsense he is saying he will move on to something else.

43

Why is it that when you try to speak or enter a conversation, others interrupt you and talk over you?

As a communication coach, I think I can answer this question with some candor. People talk over others and interrupt you for a simple but brutal fact: they don't **have social intelligence (and aren't aware of it)**.

This means that they are unable to understand when and how to intervene soberly and satisfactorily in a communicative act.

When someone talks over us we feel a sense of being overwhelmed, we see it as an extreme lack of respect for us. And in fact, to the outside eye, that's exactly what it is.

What no one ever takes into consideration though is that these people **have always interacted with others in this way**. If you've held a pen in your right hand to write since childhood, it's going to be very difficult to write with your left hand after

20 or 30 years, isn't it?

The question focuses on "why" certain people behave in a certain way and we have given a first answer: **because they have always communicated in this way.**

Going deeper, however, we must ask ourselves what drives one person to speak over another, and the answer in this case can be traced back to the classical processes of communication.

Not being used to active listening (a type of total listening, "all ears", authentic and sincere) each interlocutor is led to think of answers and things to say **even before the other finishes his part of the speech**.

A standard conversation should have this structure:

- A Enunciate (B Listen)
- B Enunciate (Link to A (Feedback) + New Element), A Listen
- A Re-work B giving feedback and adding new elements etc, etc,

This structure, which is I assure you the BASE of interpersonal communication, is never, **ever followed** (with devastating results for relationships).

This is because when A Enunciates B **is already thinking about what to say**, so he is NOT listening.

A sense of urgency is created in B precisely because he is distracted.

So what can we learn about why people talk over us? Simple, first of all they are not listening to us.

And there is no soft way to get the person to stop having this attitude.

You have to literally **verbalize what is happening**, enunciating for example *"do you know that the person talking above is not able to listen? "or "do you know what social intelligence is? It's the basis of good behavior between people, and you're breaking all the good practices by interrupting me all the time.*

I know many of you fear repercussions, but these phrases can really make your interlocutor realize that he or she is creating discomfort and could improve a lot if he or she would just be a little careful.

Because, as stated in the beginning, he or she DOES **NOT CARE!**

<h1 style="text-align:center">44</h1>

What to do when you have difficulty talking to people?

Believe it or not, the difficulty of talking to people is more prevalent than you think. So, as a coach who teaches people how to **improve their communication in the world**, I think I can give you some helpful advice to start laying the groundwork for solving this critical issue of yours.

1. **Learn to listen.** It may seem counterintuitive but listening allows you to empathize with your interlocutor, generating an authentic connection. When someone feels listened to, they have a genuine interest in learning about the opinion and life of the person in front of them. And answering questions is easier than engaging in the discussion ourselves.

2. **Reflect yourself in the other.** As long as you don't have the courage to express yourself, adapt to what the other person is saying. For example, if it's a friend with whom you have difficulty keeping the tone of a conversation high, give them "more space" and ask them questions to expand

on what they've just said, and show that you're interested. Everyone loves to talk about themselves.

3. **Communicate "your way".** I'm familiar with that feeling of shame mixed with shyness that hits us when we have to talk to people, especially if we don't know them. Any communication coach would tell you to "go for it." Not me. Engage in behaviors that make you feel comfortable and never dare to do things that aren't in your nature. Are you shy? You won't be credible in the lion's share. And that, as we'll see below, is great news.

4. **Listen to your emotions.** Never ask yourself why you're blocking, because rationally you won't be able to figure out what's blocking you. You can, however, listen to your body and the (usually primary) emotions your body suggests to you in the form of body signals. How do you feel when you need to communicate? Answer truthfully. Listen to your body, because it is never wrong.

5. **Verbalize your discomfort.** This is the most powerful advice I give my students during my coaching sessions. Like we said, you don't have to play the lion's share if you're a minnow because you won't be credible and you'll be wearing an uncomfortable mask. Just say it. As soon as you can communicate that *"you are uncomfortable talking to new people"* or that *"it is very difficult for you to start interacting with others"*. Not hiding, but rather showing our weakness allows us to create a very powerful empathic bond with the other person. The moment we verbalize we are showing awareness and we are letting our interlocutor enter an intimate zone. Precisely because of this he/she will take care of us and try to put us even more at ease. Believe it or not, the latter is a technique that even professional

speakers use to create a connection with their audience. Weird, isn't it?

The Author

My name is Emanuele (Milan, 1981) and I'm a professional trainer of Effective/Emotional Communication, Storytelling and Creativity. I live in Milan in the company of a very adorable Persian cat: Cleopatra.

My goal is to help clients and students transform the way they communicate in the world.

Focusing on communication for me means improving the dialogue we have with ourselves and others.

I offer training and growth paths characterized by a unique mix of effective communication, relational storytelling, creative thinking and studies on classic communication, emotions and social intelligence.

I've helped over 1,000 students in the classroom and over 5,000 online (through my video courses) to communicate better in business, relationships, and dialogue with the world.

I graduated in Communication (IULM) and in Entertainment and Multimedia Communication (University of Milan), and then I deepened my studies in Modern Literature (University of Milan).

In 2009 I began my career as a professional teacher and coach giving intensive courses (over 16,000 hours of lectures) at several academies in Milan.

This experience allowed me to connect with hundreds of students of all ages and backgrounds.

Each of their critical issues had as its root a communication problem.

You can get more information at https://www.emozionare.net or by writing to milanoworkshops@gmail.com

Resources

Training and Coaching

If you are interested in starting a **training course** with me visit https://www.emozionare.net. You will be able to book a free, no obligation telephone consultation.

Video Course

Discover my course (over ten hours of lessons) at https://bit.ly/3mSDBox

Some reviews of my training courses

★★★★★ A great professional! Demanding, polite, sensitive and 100% goal oriented. As a student I can say that I have found in Emanuele a mentor who is accompanying me in a delicate phase of my life. The results of the path in my case have been visible since the first lessons … my colleagues were the first to notice … I let you imagine my satisfaction!

Money well spent, his work is worth at least twice what he's asking for!

Alberto M.

★★★★★ Highly recommended! The course with Emanuele has allowed me to grow at a speed I never thought possible. He is an excellent trainer, attentive and precise. He demands a lot from his students and for this reason he always manages to bring you to the achievement of the GOALS. He doesn't work with everyone: first he needs to get to know you through an introductory phone call (he made two with me to make sure he could solve my communication problem). The phone call alone was worth the cost of 3 lessons for the advice he gave me.

What can I say, so much work, so many results!

Thank you Emanuele!

Henry C.

★★★★★ Emanuele is a serious and well-prepared teacher, always willing to help and share both his skills and his experience. Highly recommended!

Francesca A.

★★★★★ I really appreciated Emanuele's method of communication during his lessons. The plus is that he always manages to put you at ease by transmitting concepts and notions in a simple way without weighing down the lesson. Definitely recommended

Lorenzo B.

★★★★★ Emanuele is not a Superprof. He is much more: a Hyperprof, a Gigaprof. He is a father, when you are lost and have no idea which way to turn. He's a brother, when you need someone to guide you towards a destination you can't see yet. It's a friend, when you simply need someone to believe in you.

If these reasons are not enough for you…

Ivan P.

★★★★★ Emanuele is really a Superprof! I recommend him to all those who want to get involved and want to express their real potential. In addition to being competent and professional he has this gift that is very difficult to find elsewhere. He is empathetic and at the same time determined to make you give your best. He doesn't like to waste time and cares a lot about the quality of his work. What can I say, a great teacher that I would recommend to everyone! Hi Ema!

Lucia G.

★★★★★ I highly recommend working with him. Emanuele's lessons are different from all others because they are designed and customized specifically to solve your problem. He's a great professional as there are few around. From the very first meeting I noticed the difference from other trainers: you can see with the naked eye that he's a professional. Together we achieved my growth goals.

Would I trust him again?

1,000,000 times yes!

Antonio M.

★★★★★ I recommend it to everyone! Experience that I would do again 1,000 times! Working with Emanuele is stimulating and gives a lot of satisfaction! We have set the goals of our path and we have achieved them in the established time … what can I say: THANK YOU EMANUELE!

Fabio S.

★★★★★ "I contacted Emanuele via the web. I was skeptical but I realized from the first free call that I was dealing with a seasoned communications professional. He has been following me for six months and my relationship with others has improved significantly"

Francis M.

★★★★★ "The thing that amazed me most about coaching with Emanuele was seeing concrete results from the very first sessions. The exercises he assigns me every week are designed specifically to solve my problem. Thank you!"

Patrick S.

★★★★★ "When I was communicating I would freeze. Literally. Thanks to Emanuele I now feel more confident and motivated when I'm with other people. We worked out together the best strategy to 'come out of the shell' and now I feel free to express my potential!"

Lucia G.

Resources

My Books

You can find a list of all my **books** on Amazon by searching for the keyword *'Emanuele M. Barboni Dalla Costa'*.

Video Courses

Check out my **video courses** on communication and creative writing and buy them at a special price https://www.udemy.com/user/emanuelebarboni/.

Free Podcast

I post my weekly **communication** and **creativity lessons** at https://anchor.fm/podcastemozionale